The Keto Diet Cookbook For Busy People

Quick and Easy Delicious Recipes for Everyday Meals

Otis Fisher

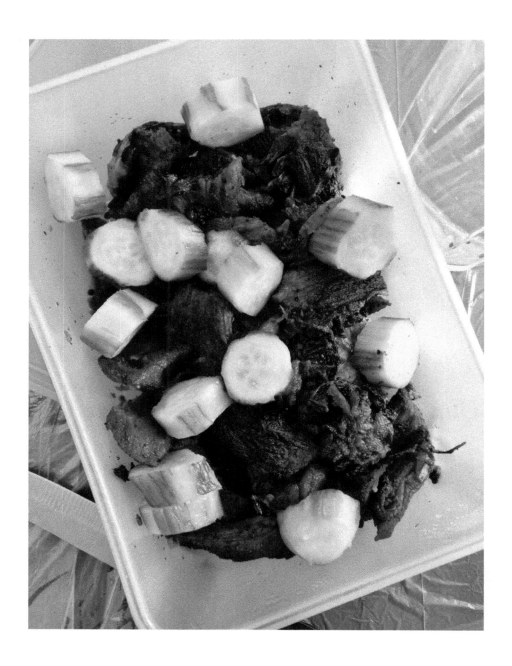

3

content within this book has been derived from various sources. Please consult a licensed professional before attempting any techniques outlined in this book.

By reading this document, the reader agrees that under no circumstances is the author responsible for any losses, direct or indirect, which are incurred as a result of the use of information contained within this document, including, but not limited to, — errors, omissions, or inaccuracies.

Table of contents

6

Cuban Pork Sandwich

Preparation Time: 5 minutes

Cooking Time: 10 minutes

Serving: 1

Ingredients:

- Sandwich Filling:
- 25 g Swiss cheese (sliced)
- 2 ounces cooked deli ham (thinly sliced)
- 3 slices pickle chips
- 1/2 tbsp. Dijon mustard
- 1/2 tbsp. mayonnaise
- 3 ounces pork roast
- 1 tsp. paprika
- 1 stalk celery (diced)

Chaffle:

- 1 tsp. baking powder
- 1 large egg (beaten)
- 1 tbsp. full-fat Greek yogurt
- 4 tbsp. mozzarella cheese
- 1 tbsp. almond flour

Directions

1. Set the oven to 350F and grease a baking sheet.
2. Plug the Chaffle maker to preheat it and spray it with a non-stick cooking spray.

3. In a mixing bowl, combine the almond flour, cheese and baking powder.

4. Add the egg and yogurt. Mix until the Ingredients: are well combined.

5. Fill the Chaffle maker with an appropriate amount of the batter and spread the batter to the edges to cover all the holes on the Chaffle maker.

6. Secure the Chaffle maker and cook the Chaffle until it is crispy. That will take about 5 minutes. The time may vary in some Chaffle makers.

7. After the cooking cycle, remove the chaffle from the Chaffle maker with a plastic or silicone utensil.

8. Repeat step 4 to 6 until you have cooked all the batter into chaffles.

9. In a small mixing bowl, merge the mustard, oregano and mayonnaise.

10. Brush the mustard-mayonnaise mixture over the surface of both chaffles.

11. Layer the pork, ham, pickles and celery over one of the chaffles. Layer the cheese slices on top and cover it with the second chaffle.

12. Place it on the baking sheet. Place it in oven and bake until the cheese melts. You can place a heavy stainless place over the chaffle to make the sandwich come out flat after baking

13. After the baking cycle, remove the chaffle sandwich from the oven and let it cool for a few minutes.

14. Serve warm and enjoy.

Nutrition:

Fat 52.3g

Carbohydrate 17.3g

Sugars 2.7g

Protein 82.6g

Turkey Chaffle Burger

Preparation Time: 5 minutes

Cooking Time: 10 minutes

Serving: 2

Ingredients:

- 2 cups ground turkey
- Salt and pepper to taste
- 1 tablespoon olive oil
- 4 garlic Chaffles
- 1 cup Romaine lettuce, chopped
- 1 tomato, sliced
- Mayonnaise
- Ketchup

Directions:

1. Combine ground turkey, salt and pepper.
2. Form thick burger patties.
3. Attach the olive oil to a pan over medium heat.
4. Cook the turkey burger until fully cooked on both sides.
5. Spread mayo on the chaffle.
6. Top with the turkey burger, lettuce and tomato.
7. Squirt ketchup on top before TOPPING with another chaffle.

Nutrition:

Calories 555

Total Fat 21.5g

Saturated Fat 3.5g

Cholesterol 117mg

Sodium 654mg

Total Carbohydrate 4.1g

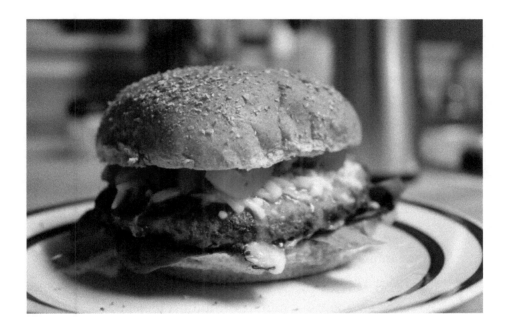

Ground Beef Chaffles

Preparation Time: 5 minutes

Cooking Time: 20 minutes

Serving: 4

Ingredients:

- 1/2 cup cooked grass-fed ground beef
- 3 cooked bacon slices, chopped
- 2 organic eggs
- 1/2 cup Cheddar cheese, shred
- 1/2 cup Mozzarella cheese, shredded
- 2 teaspoons steak seasoning

Directions:

1. Preheat a mini Chaffle iron and then grease it.
2. In a medium bowl, set all Ingredients: and mix until well combined.
3. Place 1/4 of the mixture into preheated Chaffle iron and cook for about 4-5 minutes or until golden brown.
4. Repeat with the remaining mixture.
5. Serve warm.

Nutrition:

Calories: 211

Carb: 0.g

Fat: 12g

Saturated Fat: 5.7g

Dietary Fiber: g

Sugar: 0.2g

Protein: 2.1g

Spicy Jalapeno & Bacon Chaffles

Preparation Time: 5 minutes

Cooking Time: 5 minutes

Serving: 2

Ingredients:

- 1 oz. cream cheese
- 1 large egg
- 1/2 cup cheddar cheese
- 2 tbsps. bacon bits
- 1/2 tbsp. jalapenos
- 1/4 tsp. baking powder

Directions:

1. Switch on your Chaffle maker device.
2. Set your Chaffle maker with cooking spray and let it heat up.
3. Mix together egg and vanilla extract in a bowl first.
4. Add baking powder, jalapenos and bacon bites.
5. Add in cheese last and mix together.
6. Pour the chaffles batter into the maker and cook the chaffles for about 2-3 minutes. Once chaffles are cooked, remove from the maker.
7. Serve hot and enjoy!

Nutrition:

Protein: 24

Fat: 70

Carbohydrates: 6

Savory Gruyere and Chives Chaffles

Preparation Time: 15 minutes

Cooking Time: 14 minutes

Servings: 2

Ingredients:

- 2 eggs, beaten
- 1 cup finely grated Gruyere cheese
- 2 tbsp. finely grated cheddar cheese
- 1/8 tsp. freshly ground black pepper
- 3 tbsp. minced fresh chives + more for garnishing
- 2 sunshine fried eggs for topping

Directions:

1. Preheat the Chaffle iron.
2. In a medium bowl, mix the eggs, cheeses, black pepper, and chives.
3. Open the iron and pour in half of the mixture.
4. Close the iron and Cooking until brown and crispy, 7 minutes.
5. Remove the chaffle onto a plate and set aside.
6. Make another chaffle using the remaining mixture.
7. Top each chaffle with one fried egg each, garnish with the chives and serve.

Nutrition:

Calories 712

Fats 41.32g

Protein 23.75g

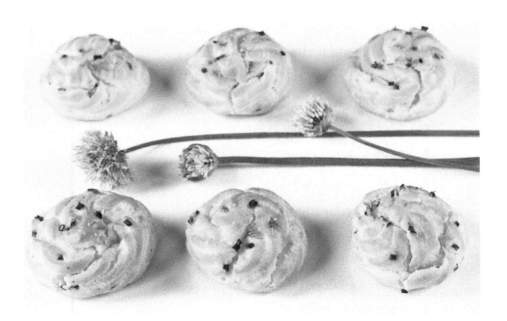

Italian Sausage Chaffles

Preparation Time: 5 minutes

Cooking Time: 8 minutes

Servings: 2

Ingredients:

- 1 egg, beaten
- 1 cup cheddar cheese, shredded
- 1/4 cup Parmesan cheese, grated
- 1 lb. Italian sausage, crumbled
- 2 teaspoons baking powder
- 1 cup almond flour

Direction:

1. Preheat your Chaffle maker.
2. Mix all the ingredients in a bowl.
3. Fill in half of the batter into the Chaffle maker.
4. Cover and Cooking for 4 minutes.
5. Transfer to a plate.
6. Let cool to make it crispy.
7. Do the same steps to make the next chaffle.

Nutrition:

Calories 332

Fat 27.1g

Protein 19.6g

LT Chaffle Sandwich

Preparation Time: 10 minutes

Cooking Time: 15 minutes

Servings: 2

Ingredients:

- Cooking spray
- 4 slices bacon
- 1 tablespoon mayonnaise
- 4 basic chaffles
- 2 lettuce leaves
- 2 tomato slices

Direction:

1. Coat your pan with foil and place it over medium heat.
2. Cooking the bacon until golden and crispy.
3. Spread mayo on top of the chaffle.
4. Top with the lettuce, bacon and tomato.
5. Top with another chaffle.

Nutrition

Calories 238

Fat 18.4g

Protein 14.3g

Sloppy Joe Chaffle

Preparation Time: 15 minutes

Cooking Time: 15 minutes

Servings: 2

Ingredients:

- 1 teaspoon olive oil
- 1 lb. ground beef
- Salt and pepper to taste
- 1 teaspoon onion powder
- 1 teaspoon garlic powder
- 3 tablespoons tomato paste
- 1 tablespoon chili powder
- 1 teaspoon mustard powder
- 1/2 teaspoon paprika
- 1/2 cup beef broth
- 1 teaspoon coconut aminos
- 1 teaspoon sweetener
- 4 cornbread chaffles

Direction:

1. Drizzle the olive oil into a pan at medium high heat.
2. Add the ground beef.
3. Season with salt, pepper and spices.
4. Cooking for 5 minutes, stirring occasionally.
5. Stir in the beef broth, coconut aminos and sweetener.
6. Reduce heat and simmer for 10 minutes.

7. Top the cornbread chaffle with the ground beef mixture.

8. Top with another chaffle.

Nutrition:

Calories 334

Fat 12.1g

Protein 48.2g

Bacon Chaffle

Preparation Time: 5 minutes

Cooking Time: 8 minutes

Servings: 2

Ingredients:

- 1 egg
- 1/2 cup cheddar cheese, shredded
- 1 teaspoon baking powder
- 2 tablespoons almond flour
- 3 tablespoons bacon bits, Cooked

Direction:

1. Turn your Chaffle maker on.
2. Beat the egg in a bowl.
3. Stir in the cheese, baking powder, almond flour and bacon bits.
4. Fill in half of the batter into the Chaffle maker.
5. Close the device.
6. Cooking for 4 minutes.
7. Open and transfer Chaffle on a plate. Let cool for 2 minutes.
8. Repeat the same procedure with the remaining batter.

Nutrition:

Calories 147

Fat 11.5 g

Protein 9.8 g

Keto Birthday Chaffle Cake

Preparation Time: 40 minutes

Cooking Time: 20 minutes

Servings: 2

Ingredients:

For Chaffle:

- Egg: 2
- Powdered sweetener: 2 tbsp.
- Cream cheese: 2 tbsp.
- Butter: 2 tbsp. (melted)
- Coconut flour: 2 tsp.
- Almond flour: 1/4 cup
- Baking powder: 1/2 tsp.
- Vanilla extract: 1/2 tsp.
- Xanthan powder 1/4 tsp.

For Frosting:

- Heavy whipping cream: 1/2 cup
- Swerve: 2 tbsp.
- Vanilla extract: 1/2 tsp.

Directions:

1. Preheat a mini Chaffle maker if needed
2. In a medium-size blender, add all the cake ingredients and blend till it forms a creamy texture
3. Let the batter sit

4. Pour the batter to the lower plate of the Chaffle maker and spread it evenly to cover the plate properly
5. Close the lid
6. Cooking for at least 4 minutes to get the desired crunch
7. Remove the chaffle from the heat and keep aside to cool totally
8. For the frosting, add all the ingredients in a bowl and use a hand mixer until the cream thickens
9. Make as many chaffles as your mixture and Chaffle maker allow
10. Frost the chaffles in a way you like
11. Serve cool and enjoy!

Nutrition

Calories 719

Fat 51.7 g

Carbs 7.3 g

Sugar 1.3 g,

Protein 56.1 g

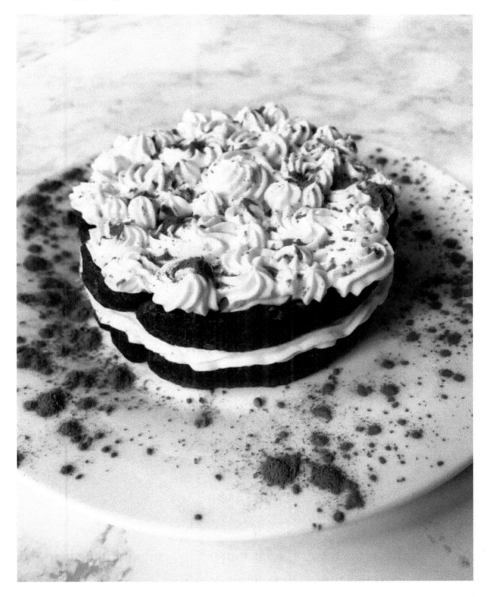

Tiramasu Chaffle Cake

Preparation Time: 20 minutes

Cooking Time: 40 minutes

Servings: 4

Ingredients:

- Egg: 2
- Monk fruit sweetener: 2 tbsp.
- Cream cheese: 2 tbsp.
- Butter: 2 tbsp. (melted)
- Coconut flour: 2 tbsp.
- Baking powder: 1 tsp.
- Vanilla extract: 1/2 tsp.
- Instant coffee dry mix: 2 1/2 tsp.
- Hazelnut extract: 1/2 tsp.
- Almond flour: 1/4 cup
- Organic cacao powder: 1 1/2 tbsp.
- Himalayan pink fine salt: 1/8 tsp.
- Mascarpone Cheese: 1/2 cup
- Powdered sweetener: 1/4 cup

Directions:

1. In a microwave, melt butter for a minute and then add instant coffee, stir it continuously
2. In a bowl, set eggs, cream cheese and the butter-coffee mixture

3. In a separate bowl, add sweetener, vanilla extract, and mascarpone cheese
4. In the egg mixture, add all the dry ingredients into it and mix well
5. Preheat a mini Chaffle maker if needed and grease it
6. Pour the egg mixture to the lower plate of the Chaffle maker and spread it evenly to cover the plate properly and close the lid
7. Cooking for at least 4 minutes to get the desired crunch
8. Remove the chaffle from the heat and keep aside to cool down
9. Make as many chaffles as your mixture and Chaffle maker allow
10. If you want to have two layers cake then split the cream
11. You can also separate cacao powder 1/2 tbsp. and instant coffee 1/2 tsp. and blend
12. Layer the cake in a way that spread cream and coffee mixture on one chaffle and add another chaffle on top
13. Serve cool and enjoy!

Nutrition

Calories 666

Fat 55.2 G

Carbs 4.8 G

Sugar 0.4 G,

Protein 37.5 G

Sodium 235 Mg

Birthday Cake Chaffle

Preparation time: 10 minutes

Cooking time: 12 minutes

Servings: 2

Ingredients:

- 1 egg (beaten)
- 2 tbsp. almond flour
- 1 tbsp. swerve sweetener
- 1/2 tsp. cake batter extract
- 1/4 tsp. baking powder
- 1 tbsp. heavy whipping cream
- 2 tbsp. cream cheese
- 1/2 tsp. vanilla extract
- 1/2 tsp. cinnamon

Frosting:

- 1 tbsp. swerve
- 1/4 cup heavy whipping cream
- 1/2 tsp. vanilla extract

Directions:

1. Plug the Chaffle maker to preheat it and spray it with a non-stick spray.
2. In a mixing bowl, combine the cinnamon, almond flour, baking powder and swerve.

3. In another mixing bowl, whisk together the egg, vanilla, heavy cream, and cake batter extract.
4. Pour the flour mixture into the egg mixture and mix until the ingredients are well combined and you have formed a smooth batter.
5. Pour an appropriate amount of the batter into the Chaffle maker and spread out the Chaffle maker to cover all the holes on the Chaffle maker.
6. Close the Chaffle maker and bake for about 3 minutes or according to your Chaffle maker's settings.
7. After the Cooking cycle, use a silicone or plastic utensil to remove the chaffle from the Chaffle maker.
8. Repeat step 5 to 7 until you have cooked all the batter into chaffles.
9. For the cream, whisk together the swerve, heavy cream and vanilla extract until smooth and fluffy.
10. To assemble the cake, place one chaffle on a flat surface and spread 1/3 of the cream over it. Layer another chaffle on the first one and spread 1/3 of the cream over it too. Repeat this for the last chaffle and the remaining cream.
11. Cut cake and serve.

Nutrition

Calories: 347

Fat: 25g

Protein: 14g

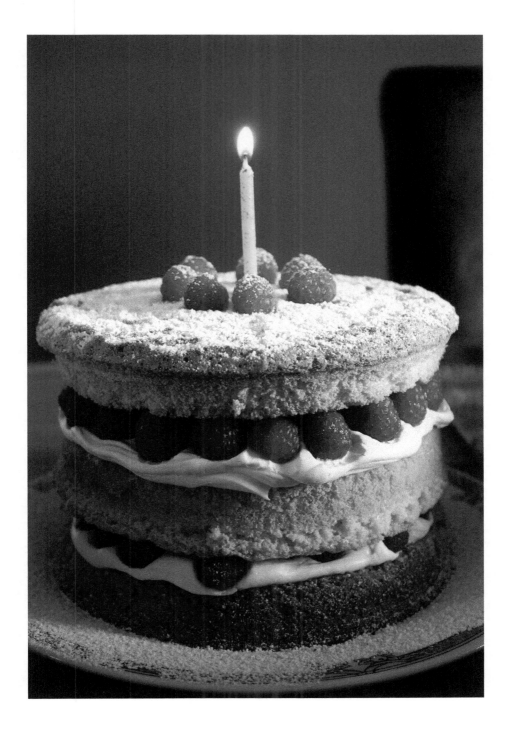

Chocolate Chaffle Cake

Preparation Time: 2 minutes

Cooking Time: 8 minutes

Servings: 2

Ingredients

- 2 tablespoons cocoa powder
- 2 tablespoons swerve granulated sugar
- 1 egg
- 1 tablespoon overwhelming whipping cream
- 1 tablespoon almond flour
- 1/2 tsp. vanilla concentrate

Directions:

1. Add all the recipes together to get the exact formula

Nutrition

Calories: 391

Fat: 21g

Protein: 14g

Keto Blueberry Chaffles

Preparation Time: 3 minutes

Cooking Time: 15 minutes

Servings: 5

Ingredients

- 1 cup of mozzarella cheddar
- 2 tablespoons almond flour
- 1 tsp. heating powder
- 2 eggs
- 1 tsp. cinnamon
- 2 tsp. of Swerve
- 3 tablespoon blueberries

Directions

1. Heat up your Dash smaller than expected Chaffle producer.
2. In a blending, bowl includes the mozzarella cheddar, almond flour, heating powder, eggs, cinnamon, swerve and blueberries. Blend well so every one of the fixings is combined.
3. Spray you're smaller than expected Chaffle producer with nonstick Cooking shower.
4. Add shortly less than 1/4 a cup of blueberry keto Chaffle player.
5. Close the top and Cook the chaffle for 3-5 minutes. Check it at the brief imprint to check whether it is firm and dark-colored. In the event that it isn't or it adheres to the highest

point of the Chaffle machine close the cover and Cooking for 1-2 minutes longer.

6. Serve with a sprinkle of swerve confectioners' sugar or keto syrup.

Nutrition:

Calories 325

Total Fat 16.3g

Protein 39.6g

Chocolate Chip Sticks

Preparation time: 10 minutes

Cooking time: 28 minutes

Servings: 4

Ingredients:

- 1 tbsp. melted butter
- 1/8 tsp. vanilla extract
- 1 tbsp. sugar-free maple syrup
- 1 egg yolk
- 1/8 tsp. baking powder
- 3 tbsp. almond flour
- 1 tbsp. unsweetened chocolate chips

Directions:

1. Preheat the Chaffle iron.
2. Attach all the ingredients to a medium bowl and mix well.
3. Open the iron and pour in a quarter of the mixture. Close the iron and Cooking until crispy, 7 minutes.
4. Remove the chaffle onto a plate and set aside.
5. Make 3 more chaffles with the remaining batter.
6. Cut the chaffles into sticks and serve.

Nutrition

Calories: 366

Fat: 27g

Protein: 10g

Sausage Ball Chaffles

Preparation time: 15 minutes

Cooking time: 28 minutes

Servings: 4

Ingredients:

- 1 lb. Italian sausage, crumbled
- 3 tbsp. almond flour
- 2 tsp. baking powder
- 1 egg, beaten
- 1/4 cup finely grated Parmesan cheese
- 1 cup finely grated cheddar cheese

Directions:

1. Preheat the Chaffle iron.
2. Set all the ingredients into a medium mixing bowl and mix well with your hands.
3. Open the iron, lightly grease with Cooking spray and add 3 tbsp. of the sausage mixture. Close the iron and Cooking for 4 minutes.
4. Open the iron; flip the chaffles and Cooking further for 3 minutes.
5. Remove the chaffle onto a plate and make 3 more using the rest of the mixture.
6. Cut each chaffle into sticks or quarters and enjoy after.

Nutrition:

Calories 132

Protein 10 g

Fat 0 g

Cholesterol 0 mg

Potassium 353 mg

Calcium 9 mg

Fiber 1.9 g

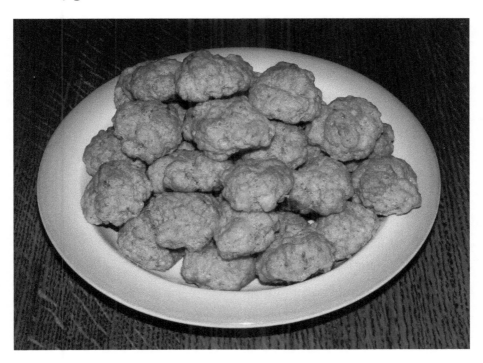

Creamy Pumpkin Pie

Preparation Time: 15 minutes

Cooking Time: 45 minutes

Servings: 6

Ingredients

For crust:

- 1 cup almond flour
- 2 tbsp. butter

For pie filling:

- 1 egg
- 1 tsp. vanilla
- 1/4 tsp. allspice
- 1/4 tsp. ground ginger
- 1/4 tsp. ground cloves
- 1 tsp. cinnamon
- 1 lemon zest
- 1/2 cup of coconut milk
- 1/2 swerve
- 1 cup pumpkin puree

Direction

1. Grease a 6-inch spring-form pan with butter and set aside.
2. Add all crust ingredients into the bowl and mix until combined.

3. Transfer crust mixture to the pan and spread evenly with the palm of your hands. Place in freezer for 15 minutes.
4. Add all filling ingredients into the food processor and process until smooth.
5. Pour filling mixture into the crust in spring-form pan.
6. Cover spring form pan with aluminum foil.
7. Pour 1 cup of water into the instant pot then place a trivet in the pot.
8. Place the pie spring-form pan on top of the trivet.
9. Seal pot with lid and select manual and set timer for 35 minutes.
10. Allow to release pressure naturally for 15 minutes then release using the quick release method.
11. Open the lid carefully. Remove pan from the pot and let it cool completely.
12. Place pie in refrigerator for 4 hours.
13. Serve chilled and enjoy.

Nutrition:

Calories 215

Fat 18.8 g

Carbohydrates 9.2 g

Sugar 2.8 g

Protein 5.9 g

Cholesterol 37 mg

Delicious Almond Peach Pie

Preparation Time: 10 minutes

Cooking Time: 15 minutes

Servings: 6

Ingredients

- 4 large eggs
- 1 tsp. lemon zest
- 1/2 tsp. vanilla
- 3 1/2 tbsp. swerve
- 1 1/2 tsp. baking powder
- 6 tbsp. butter
- 1/4 cup strawberries, chopped
- 1 medium peach, sliced
- 2 cups almond flour
- Pinch of salt

Direction

1. Grease a 7-inch cake pan with butter and line with parchment paper. Set aside.
2. In a bowl, whisk eggs with swerve. Set aside.
3. In a mixing bowl, mix together almond flour, baking powder, and salt.
4. Slowly pour almond flour mixture into the egg mixture and mix constantly.
5. Add the remaining ingredients and fold well.
6. Pour the mixture into the pan and cover the pan with foil.

7. Pour 1 cup of water into the instant pot then place a trivet in the pot.
8. Place cake pan on top of the trivet.
9. Seal instant pot with lid and select manual and set the timer for 25 minutes.
10. Release pressure using the quick release method then open the lid.
11. Remove cake pan from the pot and let it cool completely.
12. Slice and serve.

Nutrition:

Calories 380

Fat 33.6 g

Carbohydrates 12.9 g

Sugar 4.3 g

Protein 12.6 g

Cholesterol 155 mg

Creamy Chocolate Mousse

Preparation Time: 10 minutes

Cooking Time: 20 minutes

Servings: 5

Ingredients

- 4 egg yolks
- 1/2 tsp. vanilla
- 1/2 cup unsweetened almond milk
- 1 cup heavy whipping cream
- 1/4 cup unsweetened cocoa powder
- 1/4 cup of water
- 1/2 cup Swerve
- Pinch of salt

Direction

1. Add egg into a medium bowl and whisk until beaten.
2. In a saucepan, add cocoa, swerve, and water and heat over medium heat until well combined.
3. Add almond milk and cream to the pan and whisk to combine. Just heat up the mixture and remove from heat. Do not boil.
4. Add vanilla and salt and stir well.
5. Slowly pour chocolate mixture into the egg mixture and stir constantly until well combined.
6. Pour mixture into the greased ramekins.

7. Pour 2 cups of water into the instant pot then place a trivet in the pot.

8. Place ramekins on top of the trivet.

9. Seal pot with lid and select manual and set timer for 6 minutes.

10. Release pressure using the quick release method then open the lid.

11. Remove ramekins from the pot and let it cool completely.

12. Place in refrigerator for 4-6 hours.

13. Serve chilled and enjoy.

Nutrition:

Calories 141

Fat 13.4 g

Carbohydrates 3.9 g

Sugar 0.2 g

Protein 3.6 g

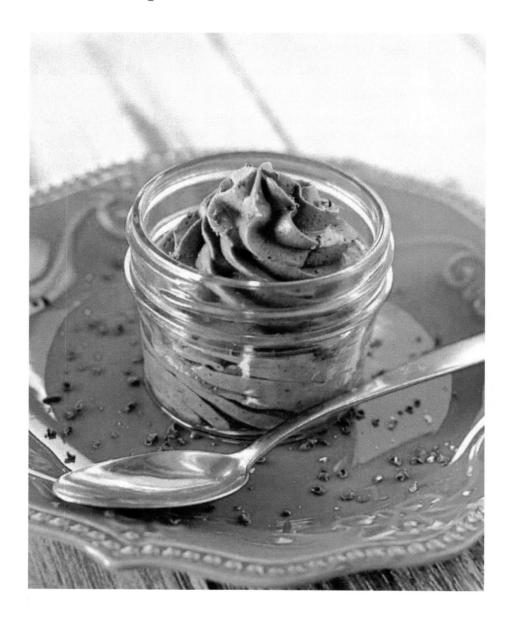

Berry Mousse

Preparation Time: 10 minutes

Cooking Time: 16 minutes

Servings: 3

Ingredients

- 1 cup strawberries, chopped
- 1 cup raspberries
- 1/4 tsp. ground ginger
- 1 tsp. vanilla
- 1/4 cup heavy cream
- 3 tbsp. whipped cream
- 1 cup unsweetened almond milk
- 1/4 cup Swerve
- Pinch of salt

Direction

1. Add berries, 1/4 cup water, and swerve into the instant pot and Cooking on sauté mode for 10-12 minutes. Stir constantly and mash lightly.
2. Once most of the liquid has evaporated from the berries mixture adds the almond milk and vanilla. Stir well and Cook for 3-4 minutes more.
3. Stir in heavy cream, whipped cream, ginger, and salt.
4. Transfer mousse mixture to the serving bowls and place in refrigerator for 3-4 hours.
5. Serve chilled and enjoy.

Nutrition:

Calories 133

Fat 9.9 g

Carbohydrates 10.4 g

Sugar 4.4 g

Protein 1.7 g

Cholesterol 30 mg

Lemon Cheesecake

Preparation Time: 10 minutes

Cooking Time: 35 minutes

Servings: 8

Ingredients

For crust:

- 2 tbsp. coconut oil, melted
- 2 tbsp. swerve
- 3/4 cup almond flour
- Pinch of salt
- For filling:
- 2 tbsp. heavy whipping cream
- 2 large eggs
- 1 tsp. lemon extract
- 1 tsp. lemon zest
- 4 tbsp. fresh lemon juice
- 2/3 cup Swerve
- 1 lb. cream cheese, softened

Direction

1. Grease a 7-inch spring-form pan with butter and line with parchment paper. Set aside.
2. In a bowl, combine together all the crust ingredients and pour into the prepared pan and spread evenly and place in refrigerator for 15 minutes.

47

3. In a large mixing bowl, beat cream cheese using a hand mixer until smooth.

4. Add swerve, lemon extract, lemon zest, and lemon juice and beat again until just combined.

5. Add eggs and heavy whipping cream and beat until well combined.

6. Pour the filling mixture over the crust and spread evenly. Cover the spring form pan with foil.

7. Pour 1 cup of water into the instant pot then place a trivet in the pot.

8. Place cake pan on top of the trivet.

9. Seal instant pot with lid and select manual high pressure for 35 minutes.

10. Allow to release pressure naturally then open the lid.

11. Remove cake pan from the pot and let it cool completely.

12. Place in refrigerator for 3-4 hours.

13. Serve chilled and enjoy.

Nutrition:

Calories 32

Fat 31.1 g

Carbohydrates 4.4 g

Sugar 0.8 g

Protein 8.3 g

Cholesterol 114 mg

Vanilla Cheesecake

Preparation Time: 10 minutes

Cooking Time: 30 minutes

Servings: 8

Ingredients

- 8 oz. cream cheese
- 2 eggs
- 1 tsp. vanilla
- 2/3 cup Swerve
- 1 cup strawberries, sliced

Direction

1. Grease a spring-form pan with butter and line with parchment paper. Set aside.
2. Add cream cheese in a large bowl and beat using a hand mixer until smooth.
3. Add vanilla and swerve and blend until well incorporated.
4. Add eggs one at a time and blend until well combined.
5. Pour batter into the pan. Cover pan tightly with foil.
6. Pour 1 cup of water into the instant pot then place a trivet in the pot.
7. Place cake pan on top of the trivet.
8. Seal instant pot with lid and select manual high pressure for 20 minutes.
9. Set to release pressure naturally for 10 minutes then release using the quick release method.

10. Open the lid carefully. Remove cake pan from the pot and let it cool completely.
11. Once the cake is completely cool then arranges strawberry slices on top of the cake.
12. Cover cake with plastic wrap and place in refrigerator overnight.
13. Serve chilled and enjoy.

Nutrition:

Calories 122

Fat 11 g

Carbohydrates 2.5 g

Sugar 1.1 g

Protein 3.6 g

Cholesterol 72 mg

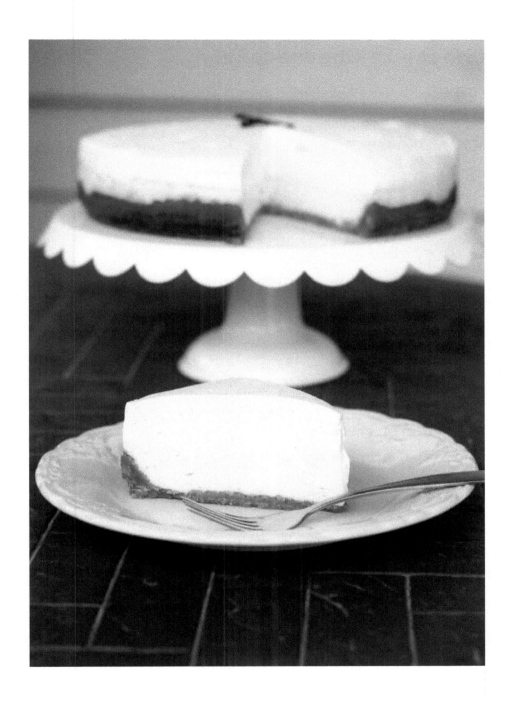

Chocolate Cheesecake

Preparation Time: 10 minutes

Cooking Time: 35 minutes

Servings: 6

Ingredients

- 16 oz. cream cheese
- 2 large eggs
- 4 tbsp. unsweetened cocoa powder
- 2 tbsp. heavy whipping cream
- 1/2 tsp. vanilla
- 2 tsp. coconut flour
- 1/2 cup Swerve
- For topping:
- 2 tsp. swerve
- 1/2 cup sour cream

Direction

1. Grease spring-form pan with butter and line with parchment paper. Set aside.
2. Add cream cheese, cocoa powder, whipping cream, vanilla, coconut flour, and swerve to the large bowl and mix until well combined using a hand mixer.
3. Add eggs one at a time and mix until well combined.
4. Pour cheesecake batter into the prepared pan.
5. Pour 1 1/2 cups of water into the instant pot then place a trivet in the pot.

6. Place cake pan on top of the trivet.
7. Seal pot with lid and Cooking on manual high pressure for 35 minutes.
8. Allow to release pressure naturally then open the lid. Remove cake pan from the pot and let it cool completely.
9. Mix together the topping ingredients and spread on top of the cake.
10. Place cake in the refrigerator for 3-4 hours.
11. Slice and serve.

Nutrition:

Calories 376

Fat 35.1 g

Carbohydrates 7.9 g

Sugar 0.8 g

Protein 9.9 g

Cholesterol 160 m

Delicious Chocó Cheesecake

Preparation Time: 10 minutes

Cooking Time: 15 minutes

Servings: 8

Ingredients

- 2 eggs
- 2 tsp. vanilla
- 1/4 cup sour cream
- 1/2 cup peanut flour
- 3/4 cup Swerve
- 16 oz. cream cheese
- 1 tbsp. coconut oil
- 1/4 cup unsweetened chocolate chips
- 2 cups of water

Direction

1. In a large bowl, beat cream cheese and swerve until smooth.
2. Gradually fold in vanilla, sour cream, and peanut flour.
3. Add eggs one at a time and fold well to combine.
4. Spray a 4-inch spring-form pan with Cooking spray.
5. Pour batter into the prepared pan and cover the pan with foil.
6. Pour 1 1/2 cups of water into the instant pot then place a trivet in the pot.
7. Place pan on top of the trivet.

8. Seal instant pot with lid and Cooking on manual high pressure for 15 minutes.
9. Allow to release pressure naturally then open the lid.
10. Remove cake pan from the pot and let it cool completely.
11. In a microwave safe bowl add coconut oil and chocolate chips and microwave for 30 seconds. Stir well.
12. Drizzle melted chocolate over the cheesecake and place in the refrigerator for 1-2 hours.
13. Serve chilled and enjoy.

Nutrition:

Calories 315

Fat 28.9 g

Carbohydrates 5.3 g

Sugar 0.3 g

Protein 8.2 g

Cholesterol 106 mg

Almond Cheesecake

Preparation Time: 10 minutes

Cooking Time: 12 minutes

Servings: 6

Ingredients

For crust:

- 3/4 cup almond flour
- 1 tsp. swerve
- 2 tbsp. butter, melted

For cake:

- 2 eggs
- 1/4 cup sour cream
- 1 tsp. vanilla
- 1/4 tsp. liquid stevia
- 8 oz. cream cheese, softened

Direction

1. Grease a 7-inch spring-form pan with butter and line with parchment paper.
2. In a bowl, combine together almond flour, butter, and swerve. Transfer crust mixture into the pan and spread evenly.
3. In another bowl beat together the liquid stevia and cream cheese until smooth.

4. Add egg one at a time. Add the sour cream and vanilla and beat until smooth.

5. Pour the cheese mixture on top of the crust and spread evenly. Cover the dish with foil.

6. Pour 2 cups of water into the instant pot and place trivet in the pot.

7. Place baking pan on top of the trivet.

8. Seal instant pot with lid and Cooking on manual high pressure for 12 minutes.

9. Allow to release pressure naturally then open the lid.

10. Remove cake pan from the pot and let it cool completely.

11. Slice and serve.

Nutrition:

Calories 290

Fat 27.5 g

Carbohydrates 5 g

Sugar 0.8 g

Protein 8 g

Cholesterol 111 mg

Ricotta Lemon Cheesecake

Preparation Time: 10 minutes

Cooking Time: 30 minutes

Servings: 6

Ingredients

- 2 eggs
- 1 lemon zest
- 1/3 cup ricotta cheese
- 1/4 cup Truvia
- 8 oz. cream cheese
- 1/2 tsp. lemon extract
- 1 lemon juice

Direction

1. Add all the ingredients except the eggs into the mixing bowl and using hand mixer blend well until no lumps.
2. Add eggs and beat until well combined.
3. Pour batter into a 6-inch spring-form pan and cover with foil.
4. Pour 2 cups of water into the instant pot and place trivet into the pot.
5. Place cake pan on top of the trivet.
6. Seal pot with lid and Cooking on high pressure for 30 minutes.
7. Allow to release pressure naturally then open the lid.

8. Remove the cake pan from the pot and let it cool completely.

9. Place in the refrigerator for 5-6 hours.

10. Serve and enjoy.

Nutrition:

Calories 178

Fat 15.8 g

Carbohydrates 6 g

Sugar 3.8 g

Protein 6.4 g

Cholesterol 100 mg

Simple Double Chicken Chaffles

Preparation Time: 5 minutes

Cooking Time: 5 minutes

Servings: 2

Ingredients:

- 1/2 cup boil shredded chicken
- 1/4 cup cheddar cheese
- 1/8 cup parmesan cheese
- 1 egg
- 1 tsp. Italian seasoning
- 1/8 tsp. garlic powder
- 1 tsp. cream cheese

Directions:

1. Preheat the Belgian Chaffle maker.
2. Mix together in chaffle ingredients in a bowl and mix together.
3. Sprinkle 1 tbsp. of cheese in a Chaffle maker and pour in chaffle batter.
4. Pour 1 tbsp. of cheese over batter and close the lid.
5. Cooking chaffles for about 4 to minutes.
6. Serve with a chicken zinger and enjoy the double chicken flavor.

Nutrition:

Calories 208

Fat 13.5g

Carbohydrate 0.7g

Protein 8.2g

Sugars 0.6g

Chaffles with Topping

Preparation Time: 5 minutes

Cooking Time: 10 minutes

Servings: 3

Ingredients:

- 1 large egg
- 1 tbsp. almond flour
- 1 tbsp. full-fat Greek yogurt
- 1/8 tsp. baking powder
- 1/4 cup shredded Swiss cheese
- TOPPING
- 4oz. grill prawns
- 4 oz. steamed cauliflower mash 1/2 zucchini sliced
- 3 lettuce leaves
- 1 tomato, sliced
- 1 tbsp. flax seeds

Directions:

1. Make 3 chaffles with the given chaffles ingredients.
2. For serving, arrange lettuce leaves on each chaffle.
3. Top with zucchini slice, grill prawns, cauliflower mash and a tomato slice.
4. Drizzle flax seeds on top.
5. Serve and enjoy!

Nutrition:

Calories 208

Fat 13.5g

Carbohydrate 0.7g

Protein 8.2g

Sugars 0.6g

Chaffle with Cheese and Bacon

Preparation Time: 5 minutes

Cooking Time: 15 minutes

Servings: 2

Ingredients:

- 1 egg
- 1/2 cup cheddar cheese, shredded
- 1 tbsp. parmesan cheese
- 3/4 tsp. coconut flour
- 1/4 tsp. baking powder
- 1/8 tsp. Italian Seasoning
- pinch of salt
- 1/4 tsp. garlic powder

For Topping

- 1 bacon sliced, Cooked and chopped
- 1/2 cup mozzarella cheese, shredded
- 1/4 tsp. parsley, chopped

Directions:

1. Preheat oven to 400 degrees.
2. Switch on your Chaffle maker and grease with Cooking spray.
3. Mix together chaffle ingredients in a mixing bowl until combined.

4. Spoon half of the batter in the center of the Chaffle maker and close the lid. Cooking chaffles for about 3-minutes until Cooked.
5. Carefully remove chaffles from the maker.
6. Arrange chaffles in a greased baking tray.
7. Top with mozzarella cheese, chopped bacon and parsley.
8. And bake in the oven for 4 -5 minutes.
9. Once the cheese is melted, remove from the oven.
10. Serve and enjoy!

Nutrition:

Calories 208

Fat 13.5g

Carbohydrate 0.7g

Protein 8.2g

Sugars 0.6g

Grill Beefsteak and Chaffle

Preparation Time: 5 minutes

Cooking Time: 10 minutes

Servings: 1

Ingredients:

- 1 beefsteak rib eye
- 1 tsp. salt
- 1 tsp. pepper
- 1 tbsp. lime juice
- 1 tsp. garlic

Directions:

1. Prepare your grill for direct heat.
2. Mix together all spices and rub over beefsteak evenly.
3. Set the beef on the grill rack over medium heat.
4. Secure and Cooking steak for about6 to 8 minutes. Flip and Cooking for another 5 minutes until Cooked through.
5. Serve with keto simple chaffle and enjoy!

Nutrition:

Calories 208

Fat 13.5g

Carbohydrate 0.7g

Protein 8.2g

Sugars 0.6g

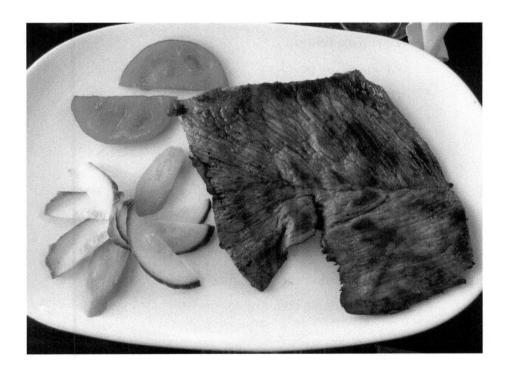

Cauliflower Chaffles and Tomatoes

Preparation Time: 5 minutes

Cooking Time: 15 minutes

Servings: 2

Ingredients:

- 1/2 cup cauliflower
- 1/4 tsp. garlic powder
- 1/4 tsp. black pepper
- 1/4 tsp. Salt
- 1/2 cup shredded cheddar cheese
- 1 egg

For Topping

- 1 lettuce leave
- 1 tomato sliced
- 4 oz. cauliflower steamed, mashed
- 1 tsp. sesame seeds

Directions:

1. Add all chaffle ingredients into a blender and mix well.
2. Sprinkle 1/8 shredded cheese on the Chaffle maker and pour cauliflower mixture in a preheated Chaffle maker and sprinkle the rest of the cheese over it.
3. Cooking chaffles for about 4-5 minutes until Cooked
4. For serving, lay lettuce leaves over chaffle top with steamed cauliflower and tomato.
5. Drizzle sesame seeds on top.

6. Enjoy!

Nutrition:

Calories 208

Fat 13.5g

Carbohydrate 0.7g

Protein 8.2g

Sugars 0.6g

Jicama Loaded Baked Potato Chaffle

Preparation time: 5 minutes

Cooking time: 5 minutes

Servings: 2

Ingredients

- 1 big jicama root
- 1/2 medium onion
- 2 garlic cloves
- 1 cup cheese of choice
- 2 eggs whisked
- Salt and pepper

Directions:

1. Put jicama shredded in a large colander, sprinkle with 1-2 tsp. of salt. Mix well and drain well.
2. Microwave for 5-8 minutes.
3. Mix all ingredients.
4. Whisk a little cheese on Chaffle iron before adding 3 T of the mixture; sprinkle a little more cheese on top of the Cooking mixture for 5 minutes.
5. Two more flip and fry.
6. Top with a dollop of sour cream, pieces of bacon cheese and peppers!

Nutrition:

Calories 168 Kcal

Total Fat 11.8g

Cholesterol 121mg

Sodium 221.8mg

Total Carbohydrate 5.1g

Dietary Fiber 1.7g

Sugars 1.2g

Protein 10g

Oreo Cookies Chaffle

Preparation time: 5 minutes

Cooking time: 5 minutes

Servings: 3

Ingredients

Chaffle ingredients:

- 1 egg
- 1 cup of black cocoa
- 1 tbs. monk fruit confectioners blend or favorite keto-approved sweetener
- 1/4 teaspoon baking powder
- Cream cheese 2 room temperature, softened at room temperature
- 1 tablespoon of mayonnaise
- 1/4 teaspoon non-liquid instant coffee powder
- Pinch salt
- 1 teaspoon of vanilla
- Matting ingredient:
- 2 Tbs. monk fruit confectionery
- 2 Tbs. cream cheese softens, room temperature
- 1/4 teaspoon transparent vanilla

Directions:

1. Attach the rest of the ingredients and mix well until smooth and creamy.

2. Divide the batter into 3 and pour each into a mini Chaffle maker and Cooking until it is fully cooked for 2 1/2 to 3 minutes.

3. Add the sweetener, cream cheese, and vanilla in a separate small bowl. Mix the frosting until all is well embedded.

4. Whisk the frosting on the cake after it has cooled down to room temperature.

Nutrition:

Calories 69 Kcal

Total Fat 5g

Cholesterol 67.4mg

Sodium 874.7mg

Total Carbohydrate 2.7g

Dietary Fiber 0.7g

Sugars 0.9g

Protein 3.5g

Best Keto Chaffle

Preparation time: 10 minutes

Cooking time: 5 minutes

Servings: 4

Ingredients

- 2 eggs
- 1 cup shredded cheddar cheese
- 1 Scoop Perfect Keto Flavored Collagen

Directions:

1. Warmth the mini Chaffle iron.
2. While the Chaffle iron is heating, merge all ingredients in a medium-sized bowl.
3. Spoon 1/4 cup of mix into Chaffle maker and Cooking for 3-4 minutes or until Chaffles are crisp.
4. Serve and enjoy!

Nutrition:

Calories: 326 Kcal

Fat: 24.75g

Carbohydrates: 2g (net: 1g)

Fiber: 1g

Protein: 25g

Keto Chaffle Churro

Preparation time: 10 minutes

Cooking time: 4 minutes

Servings: 2

Ingredients:

- 1 egg
- 1/2 cup mozzarella cheese shredded
- 2 tbsp. swallow brown sweetener
- 1/2 tsp. cinnamon

Directions:

1. Preheat the mini Chaffle of iron.
2. Whip the egg in a bowl.
3. Apply the shredded cheese to the combination of eggs.
4. Place half of the egg mixture in a mini Chaffle pan and Cooking until golden brown
5. Once the Chaffle is done, cut it into slices. Serve warm and enjoy!

Nutrition:

Calories 76 Kcal

Total Fat 4.3g

Cholesterol 14mg

Sodium 147.5mg

Total Carbohydrate 4.1g

Dietary Fiber 1.2g

Sugars 1.9g

Protein 5.5g

Keto Zucchini Toast

Preparation Time: 15 minutes

Cooking Time: 20 minutes

Servings: 4

Ingredients

- 1/4 cup almond flour
- 1 cup zucchini, shredded and boiled
- 1/4 tsp. garlic powder
- 1 egg
- 1 Tbsp. flax meal
- 1 pinch black pepper
- 1/4 tsp. oregano
- 1 pinch salt
- 1/4 tsp. basil

Directions

1. Set the oven to 450F and line a baking sheet with parchment paper.
2. Whisk the eggs with the rest of the ingredients in a bowl to form a batter.
3. Divide the batter into 4 equal parts and lay each on the baking sheet.
4. Transfer the sheet to the oven and bake for 20 minutes.
5. Remove, cool, and serve.

Nutrition:

Calories: 71

Fat: 5.1g

Carb: 3.2g

Protein: 3.6g

Protein Keto Bread

Preparation Time: 10 minutes

Cooking Time: 40 minutes

Servings: 12

Ingredients:

- 1/2 cup unflavored protein powder
- 6 tbsp. almond flour
- 5 pastured eggs, separated
- 1 tbsp. coconut oil
- 1 tsp. baking powder
- 1 tsp. xanthan gum
- 1 pinch Himalayan pink salt
- 1 pinch stevia (optional)

Directions:

1. Begin by setting the oven to 325 degrees F.
2. Grease a ceramic loaf dish with coconut oil and layer it with parchment paper.
3. Add egg whites to a bowl and beat well until it forms peaks.
4. In a separate bowl, mix the dry ingredients.
5. Mix wet ingredients in another bowl and beat well.
6. Fold in dry mixture and mix well until smooth.
7. Fold in the egg whites and mix evenly.
8. Spread the bread batter in the prepared loaf pan.
9. Bake the bread for 40 minutes or until it's done.
10. Slice into 12 slices and serve.

Nutrition:

Cal: 165

Total Fat 14 g

Saturated Fat 7 g

Cholesterol 632 mg

Sodium 497 mg

Total Carbs 6 g

Fiber 3 g

Sugar 1 g

Protein 5 g

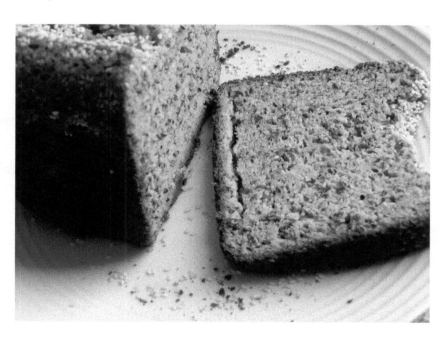

Keto Breakfast Bread

Preparation Time: 15 minutes

Cooking Time: 40 minutes

Servings: 16 slices

Ingredients:

- 1/2 tsp. xanthan gum
- 1/2 tsp. salt
- 2 Tbsp. coconut oil
- 1/2 cup butter, melted
- 1 tsp. baking powder
- 2 cups of almond flour
- 7 eggs

Directions:

1. Preheat the oven to 355F.
2. Beat eggs in a bowl on high for 2 minutes.
3. Add coconut oil and butter to the eggs and continue to beat.
4. Line a loaf pan with baking paper and pour the beaten eggs.
5. Pour in the rest of the ingredients and mix until it becomes thick.
6. Bake until a toothpick comes out dry, about 40 to 45 minutes.

Nutrition:

Calories: 234

Fat: 23g

Carb: 1g

Protein: 7g

Almond Keto Bread

Preparation Time: 10 minutes

Cooking Time: 30 minutes

Servings: 10

Ingredients:

- 1 1/2 cup almond flour
- 6 large eggs, separated
- 1/4 cup butter, melted
- 3 tsp. baking powder
- 1/4 tsp. cream of tartar
- 1 pinch pink Himalayan salt
- 6 drops liquid stevia

Directions:

1. Start by your oven to 375 degrees F.
2. Now, separate the egg yolks from their whites.
3. Beat the whites with cream of tartar in a mixing bowl until it's foamy and creamy.
4. Blend egg yolks with butter, almond flour, salt, baking powder, stevia, and 1/3 of the egg white mixture in a food processor.
5. Once blended well, fold in the remaining egg whites, and then transfer the batter to a greased 8x4 loaf pan.
6. Bake the bread for 30 minutes or until it's done.
7. Slice into 20 slices and serve fresh.

Nutrition:

Cal: 107

Total Fat: 9.3 g

Saturated Fat: 4.8 g

Cholesterol: 77 mg

Sodium 135 mg

Total Carbs 2.6 g

Fiber 0.8 g

Sugar 9.9 g

Protein 3.9 g

Buttery Bagels

Preparation Time: 10 minutes

Cooking Time: 23 minutes

Servings: 6

Ingredients:

- 1/2 tsp. baking soda
- 1 3/4 Tbsp. butter, unsalted and melted
- 3 eggs, separated
- 1/4 tsp. cream of tartar
- 2 Tbsp. coconut flour, sifted
- 1 3/4 Tbsp. cream cheese, full-fat and softened
- 2 tsp. Swerve sweetener, granulated
- 1/4 tsp. salt
- Coconut oil Cooking spray

Directions:

1. Preheat the oven to 300F. Coat a 6-cavity donut pan with coconut oil spray.
2. Divide the eggs between whites and yolks.
3. Blend the cream of tartar with the egg whites and pulse with a hand mixer for 5 minutes.
4. Combine the egg yolks with salt, baking soda, Swerve, coconut flour, melted butter, and cream cheese.
5. Gently blend the whipped eggs into the mix and blend well.
6. Fill the pan with the batter.
7. Bake in the oven for 23 minutes.

8. Cool and serve.

Nutrition:

Calories: 83

Fat: 3g

Carb: 1.2g

Protein: 6g

Psyllium Husk Bread

Preparation Time: 10 minutes

Cooking Time: 35 minutes

Servings: 10

Ingredients:

- 1/2 cup coconut flour
- 2 tbsp. psyllium husk powder
- 1/2 tsp. baking powder
- 1/4 tsp. pink Himalayan salt
- 3/4 cup water
- 4 large eggs
- 4 tbsp. butter

Directions:

1. Start by whisking the husk powder, salt, baking powder, and coconut flour in a bowl.
2. Beat eggs with water and melted butter in a mixer until its smooth.
3. Slowly stir in the dry mixture and mix well until smooth.
4. Make 10 dinner rolls out of this bread dough and place the dough on a baking sheet.
5. Bake them for 35 minutes, approximately, at 350 degrees F until all done.
6. Slice and serve.

Nutrition:

Cal: 220

Total Fat: 20.1 g

Saturated Fat: 7.4 g

Cholesterol: 132 mg

Sodium: 157 mg

Total Carbs: 63 g

Sugar: 0.4 g

Fiber: 2.4 g

Protein: 6.1 g

Coconut Cloud Bread

Preparation Time: 10 minutes

Cooking Time: 25 minutes

Servings: 4

Ingredients:

- 3 eggs
- 3 tbsp. coconut cream
- 1/2 tsp. baking powder
- Optional toppings:
- sea salt
- black pepper
- rosemary

Directions:

1. First, set aside the egg yolks and egg whites.
2. Beat egg yolks in a bowl.
3. Stir in cream and continue beating with a hand mixer until creamy and smooth.
4. Beat the egg whites with baking powder in another bowl until it forms peaks.
5. Quickly add yolk mixture to the whites and mix well until fluffy.
6. Spread 1/4 of the batter onto a baking sheet separately to make 4 circles.
7. Bake the batter for 25 minutes approximately at 350 degrees F.

8. Serve.

Nutrition:

Cal: 158

Total Fat: 15.2 g

Saturated Fat: 5.2 g

Cholesterol 269 mg

Sodium 178 mg

Total Carbs 7.4 g

Sugar 1.1 g

Fiber 3.5 g

Protein 5.5 g

Macadamia Nut Bread

Preparation Time: 10 minutes

Cooking Time: 40 minutes

Servings: 6

Ingredients:

- 5 oz. macadamia nuts
- 5 large eggs
- 1/4 cup coconut flour
- 1/2 tsp. baking soda
- 1/2 tsp. apple cider vinegar

Directions:

1. Begin by placing the oven to 350 degrees F.
2. Blend macadamia nuts in a food processor until it forms nut butter.
3. Continue blending while adding eggs one by one until well incorporated.
4. Stir in apple cider vinegar, baking soda, and coconut flour.
5. Blend until well mixed and incorporated.
6. Set a bread pan with Cooking spray and spread the batter in a pan.
7. Bake the batter for 40 minutes approximately until golden brown.
8. Slice and serve.

Nutrition:

Cal: 248

Total Fat: 19.3 g

Saturated Fat: 4.8 g

Cholesterol: 32 mg

Sodium: 597 mg

Total Carbs: 3.1 g

Fiber: 0.6 g

Sugar: 1.9 g

Protein: 7.9 g

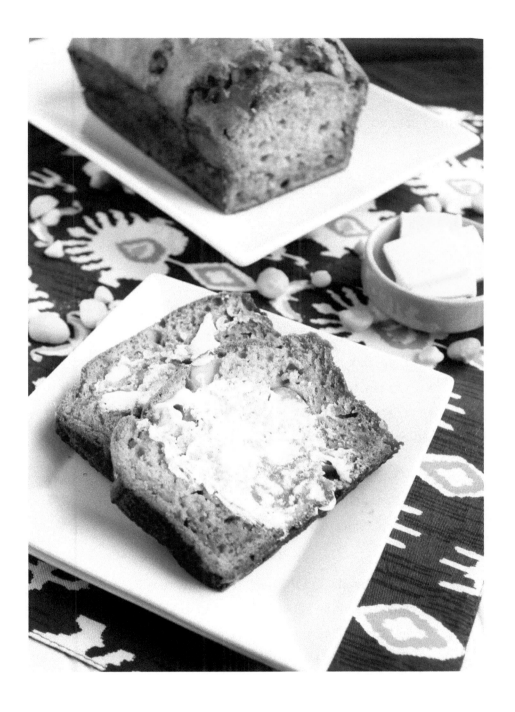

Garlic Focaccia Bread

Preparation Time: 10 minutes

Cooking Time: 20 minutes

Servings: 4

Ingredients:

Dry Ingredients

- 1 cup almond flour
- 1/4 cup coconut flour
- 1/2 tsp. xanthan gum
- 1 tsp. garlic powder
- 1 tsp. flaky salt
- 1/2 tsp. baking soda
- 1/2 tsp. baking powder

Wet Ingredients

- 2 eggs
- 1 tbsp. lemon juice
- 2 tsp. olive oil + 2 tbsp. olive oil to drizzle

Directions:

1. Begin by placing the oven to 350 degrees F.
2. Layer a baking sheet with parchment paper.
3. Now, whisk all the dry ingredients in a bowl.
4. Beat lemon juice, oil, and egg in a bowl until well incorporated.
5. Whisk in dry ingredients and mix well until it forms dough.

6. Bring the dough on a baking sheet and cover it with aluminum foil.

7. Bake for 10 minutes approximately then remove the foil.

8. Drizzle olive oil on top and bake for another 10 minutes uncovered.

9. Garnish with basil and Italian seasoning.

10. Serve.

Nutrition:

Cal: 301

Total Fat: 26.3 g

Saturated Fat: 14.8 g

Cholesterol: 322 mg

Sodium: 597 mg

Total Carbs: 2.6 g

Fiber: 0.6 g

Sugar: 1.9 g

Protein: 12 g

Cauliflower Bread

Preparation Time: 10 minutes

Cooking Time: 54 minutes

Servings: 8

Ingredients:

- 3 cup cauliflower rice
- 10 large egg
- 1/4 tsp. cream of tartar
- 1 1/4 cup coconut flour
- 1 1/2 tbsp. gluten-free baking powder
- 1 tsp. sea salt
- 6 tbsp. butter
- 6 cloves garlic (minced)
- 1 tbsp. fresh rosemary (chopped)
- 1 tbsp. fresh parsley (chopped)

Directions:

1. Begin by starting the oven to 350 degrees F and layer a loaf pan with parchment paper.
2. Place the cauliflower rice in a large bowl and cover it with a plastic sheet.
3. Cooking the rice in the microwave for 4 minutes.
4. During this time, beat egg whites with cream of tartar in a bowl until it forms peaks.
5. Whisk coconut flour with egg yolks, salt, baking powder, garlic, and melted butter in a separate bowl.

6. Stir in 1/4 egg whites and blend the mixture in a food processor until incorporated.
7. Set the cauliflower rice in a kitchen towel and squeeze to absorb moisture from the rice.
8. Add the cauliflower rice to the food processor and pulse until well mixed.
9. Fold in rosemary and parsley.
10. Spread the cauliflower batter in a baking pan lined with parchment paper.
11. Bake the batter for 50 minutes until golden brown.
12. Slice and serve fresh.

Nutrition:

Cal: 282

Total Fat: 25.1 g

Saturated Fat: 8.8 g

Cholesterol: 100 mg

Sodium: 117 mg

Total Carbs: 9.4 g

Sugar: 0.7 g

Fiber: 3.2 g

Protein: 8 g

Buttery Flatbread

Preparation Time: 10 minutes

Cooking Time: 8 minutes

Servings: 4

Ingredients:

1 cup almond flour

2 tbsp. coconut flour

2 tsp. xanthan gum

1/2 tsp. baking powder

1/2 tsp. flaky salt

1 whole egg + 1 egg white

1 tbsp. water

1 tbsp. oil, for frying

1 tbsp. melted butter, for slathering

Directions:

1. Start by whisking baking powder, salt, flour, and xanthan gum in a bowl.
2. Beat egg whites and egg in a bowl until creamy.
3. Fold in flour mixture and mix until well incorporated.
4. Add a tablespoon of water to the dough and cut it into 4 equal parts.

5. Spread each part out into a flatbread and Cooking each for 1 minute per side in a skillet with oil.
6. Garnish with butter, parsley, and salt.
7. Serve.

Nutrition:

Cal: 216

Total: Fat: 20.9 g

Saturated Fat: 8.1 g

Cholesterol: 241 mg

Total Carbs: 8.3 g

Sugar: 1.8 g

Fiber: 3.8 g

Sodium: 8 mg

Protein: 6.4 g

Keto Yeast Loaf Bread

Preparation Time: 5 minutes

Cooking Time: 4 hours

Total Time: 4 hours 5 minutes

Servings: 16 slices

Ingredients:

- 1 package dry yeast
- 1/2 tsp. sugar
- 1 1/8 cup warm water about 90-100 degrees F
- 3 tbsps. Olive oil or avocado oil
- 1 cup vital wheat gluten flour
- 1/4 cup oat flour
- 3/4 cup soy flour
- 1/4 cup flax meal
- 1/4 cup wheat bran course, unprocessed
- 1 tbsp. sugar
- 1 1/2 tsp. baking powder
- 1 tsp. salt

Directions:

1. Merge the sugar, water, and yeast in the bread bucket to proof the yeast. If the yeast does not bubble, toss and replace it.

2. Combine all the dry ingredients in a bowl and mix thoroughly. Pour over the wet ingredients in the bread bucket.

3. Set the bread machine and select BASIC cycle to bake the loaf. Close the lid. This takes 3 to 4 hours.

4. When the cycle ends, remove the bread from the bread machine.

5. Cool on a rack before slicing.

6. Serve with butter or light jam.

Nutrition:

Cal: 99

Calories from fat: 45

Total Fat: 5 g

Total Carbohydrates: 7 g

Net Carbohydrates: 5 g

Protein: 9 g

Creamy Bacon Salad on a Chaffle

Preparation Time: 5 minutes

Cooking Time: 15 minutes

Serving: 4

Ingredients:

- 4 eggs
- 11/2 cups grated mozzarella cheese
- 1/2 cup parmesan cheese
- Salt and pepper to taste
- 1 teaspoon dried oregano
- 1/4 cup almond flour
- 2 teaspoons baking powder

Bacon salad

- 1/2 pound Cooked bacon
- 1 cup cream cheese
- 1 teaspoon dried oregano
- 1 teaspoon dried basil
- 1 teaspoon dried rosemary
- 2 tablespoons lemon juice

Other

- 2 tablespoons butter to brush the Chaffle maker
- 2 spring onions, finely chopped, for serving

Directions

1. Preheat the Chaffle maker.

2. Add the eggs, mozzarella cheese, parmesan cheese, salt and pepper, dried oregano, almond flour and baking powder to a bowl.
3. Mix until combined.
4. Brush the heated Chaffle maker with butter and add a few tablespoons of the batter.
5. Close the lid and Cooking for about 5–7 minutes depending on your Chaffle maker.
6. Meanwhile, chop the cooked bacon into smaller pieces and place them in a bowl with the cream cheese. Season with dried oregano, dried basil, dried rosemary and lemon juice.
7. Mix until combined and spread each chaffle with the creamy bacon salad.
8. To serve, sprinkle some freshly chopped spring onion on top.

Nutrition

Calories 750

Fat 62.5 g

Carbs 7.7 g

Sugar 0.8 g,

Protein 40.3 g

Sodium 1785 Mg

Mediterranean Lamb Kebabs on Chaffle

Preparation Time: 5 minutes

Cooking Time: 15 minutes

Serving: 4

Ingredients:

- 4 eggs
- 2 cups grated mozzarella cheese
- Salt and pepper to taste
- 1 teaspoon garlic powder
- 1/4 cup Greek yogurt
- 1/2 cup coconut flour
- 2 teaspoons baking powder

Lamb kebabs

- 1 pound ground lamb meat
- Salt and pepper to taste
- 1 egg
- 2 tablespoons almond flour
- 1 spring onion, finely chopped
- 1/2 teaspoon dried garlic
- 2 tablespoons olive oil

Other

- 2 tablespoons butter to brush the Chaffle maker
- 1/4 cup sour cream for serving

- 4 sprigs of fresh dill for garnish

Directions

1. Preheat the Chaffle maker.
2. Add the eggs, mozzarella cheese, salt and pepper, garlic powder, Greek yogurt, coconut flour and baking powder to a bowl.
3. Mix until combined.
4. Brush the heated Chaffle maker with butter and add a few tablespoons of the batter.
5. Close the lid and Cooking for about 5–7 minutes depending on your Chaffle maker.
6. Meanwhile, add the ground lamb, salt and pepper, egg, almond flour, chopped spring onion, and dried garlic to a bowl. Mix and form medium-sized kebabs.
7. Impale each kebab on a skewer. Warmth the olive oil in a frying pan.
8. Cooking the lamb kebabs for about 3 minutes on each side.
9. Serve each chaffle with a tablespoon of sour cream and one or two lamb kebabs. Decorate with fresh dill.

Nutrition

Calories 679

Fat 49.9 G

Carbs 15.8 G

Sugar 0.8 G,

Protein 42.6 G,

Sodium 302 Mg

Lamb Chops on Chaffle

Preparation Time: 5 minutes

Cooking Time: 20 minutes

Serving: 4

Ingredients:

- 4 eggs
- 2 cups grated mozzarella cheese
- Salt and pepper to taste
- 1 teaspoon garlic powder
- 1/4 cup heavy cream
- 6 tablespoons almond flour
- 2 teaspoons baking powder

Lamb chops

- 2 tablespoons herbed butter
- 1 pound lamb chops
- Salt and pepper to taste
- 1 teaspoon freshly chopped rosemary

Other

- 2 tablespoons butter to brush the Chaffle maker
- 2 tablespoons freshly chopped parsley for garnish

Directions

1. Preheat the Chaffle maker.

2. Add the eggs, mozzarella cheese, salt and pepper, garlic powder, heavy cream, almond flour and baking powder to a bowl.
3. Mix until combined.
4. Brush the heated Chaffle maker with butter and add a few tablespoons of the batter.
5. Close the lid and Cooking for about 5–7 minutes depending on your Chaffle maker.
6. Meanwhile, heat a nonstick frying pan and rub the lamb chops with herbed butter, salt and pepper, and freshly chopped rosemary.
7. Cooking the lamb chops for about 3–4 minutes on each side.
8. Serve each chaffle with a few lamb chops and sprinkle on some freshly chopped parsley for a nice presentation.

Nutrition

Calories 537

Fat 37.3 g

Carbs 5.5 g

Sugar 0.6 g,

Protein 44.3 g

Sodium 328 Mg